MW01017152

Anti Inflammatory Diet:

Beginner's Guide: What You Need to Know to Heal Yourself with Food + Recipes + One Week Diet Plan

Copyright © 2014 by Annette Goodman

All rights reserved. No part of this publication may be reproduced, stored in a retrieval system, or transmitted, in any form or by any means, electronic, mechanical, photocopying, recording or otherwise without the prior written permission of the author and the publishers.

All information in this book has been carefully researched and checked for factual accuracy. However, the author and publishers make no warranty, expressed or implied, that the information contained herein is appropriate for every individual, situation or purpose and assume no responsibility for errors and omission.

Under no circumstances should be the advice included in this book treated as a medical consultation substitute. Before applying any dietary change, the reader should agree it with their doctor first. The reader assumes the risk and full responsibility for all actions, and the author will not be held liable for any loss or damage, whether consequential, incidental, and special or otherwise that may result from the information presented in this publication.

Table of Contents:

@

My Mailing list: If you would like to **receive new Kindle reads** on **weight loss, wellness, diets, recipes and healthy living** for **FREE** I invite you to my Mailing List. Whenever my new book is out, I set the free period for two days. You will get an e-mail notification and will **be the first to get the book for $0** during its limited promotion.

Why would I do this when it took me countless hours to write these e-books?

First of all, that's my way of saying **"thank you"** to my new readers. Second of all – **I want to spread the word about my new books and ideas.** Mind you that **I hate spam and e-mails that come too frequently** - no worries about that.

If you think that's a good idea and are in, just follow this link:

http://eepurl.com/6elQD

Anti Inflammatory Diet: Beginner's Guide

Introduction

Hello Friends!

Thank you for choosing this book!

A proper plan and its follow-up can immensely help to reach the stipulated targets, especially when you are trying to fight a problem as aggressive and as common as inflammation. This book covers all the essentials of what an anti-inflammatory diet should contain, and tells you how to use the perfect combination of ingredients, fruits and vegetables for the best results.

The diet is packed with a variety in terms of what you can eat and is mainly comprised of fresh foods. In addition to this, it contains a lot of fresh fruits and vegetables. On the other hand, it emphasizes cutting out processed or packaged foods. The diet has a perfect balance of carbohydrates, fats and proteins, which ensures an optimum balance of calories, thereby controlling weight and preventing its fluctuation.

Use this book as your perfect guide to achieve the desired results and start your journey to staying healthy and fit!

Chapter 1: Understanding the Anti-Inflammatory Diet

Excess inflammation has always been a cause for concern. Sadly, it has not garnered the attention it deserves. Unchecked and unrestrained, it can lead to asthma, allergies, tissue and cell degeneration, heart diseases, cancer and various other maladies, which are difficult to deal with. The sad fact remains that once infected with inflammation, usually no medicine or conventional medical treatments will yield the desired result.

Chronic inflammation damages the body and leads to many diseases and illnesses, negatively impacting the immunity of our body. This can have serious repercussions in the long run. Therefore, it becomes an absolute necessity to deal with these at their onset. Correct dietary choices can prove to be very helpful in the long run to deal with these issues. An anti-inflammatory diet has a scientific basis to it and is thereby a long-term plan focused on a healthy body. It is aimed at providing energy to the body and consists of vitamins, minerals, nutrients and essential fatty acids.

The anti-inflammatory diet can keep heart diseases at bay, check cardiovascular problems, reduce blood pressure, check arthritis and other bone issues, thereby ensuring an agile body capable of fighting diseases and increasing your immunity. Inflammation has acquired much attention in recent years because of the serious threat it poses in the facilitation of certain ailments. It works silently and is said to be the trigger for many maladies. An anti-inflammatory diet, which is also in many ways similar to a Mediterranean diet, emerges as a perfect diet plan that must be adopted in order to deal with these maladies.

The anti-inflammatory diet does not come with vague promises of doing wonders for you in the blink of an eye. In fact, it is unlike any of those crash diets that are in vogue these days, especially among youngsters who are ready to trade off anything for a fit and fabulous body.

Contrary to popular belief, an anti-inflammatory diet can be considered a plan for life. An anti-inflammatory diet is comprised of healthy, tasty and wholesome foods that are unprocessed. It is a diet that can be considered an ideal diet for dealing with numerous diseases and is said to provide good health.

Testimony

I myself suffered from long and gruesome periods of acute inflammation. I had IBS symptoms and very bad, extremely painful sinusitis. It started to affect my day-to-day ability to work, and my potential and productivity suffered a steep decline. Medication helped, but the effect was only temporary. The fact that I was slightly overweight did not help either. I would be confined to my house for days without any solution to my problem. Every doctor I visited could pinpoint the superficial problem and treat it, time after time, but none could tell me what was causing this problem.

Having faced enough failure to look for a solution, I decided to do a bit of my own research. I read a plethora of material on the anti-inflammatory diet and filtered fact from fiction. Then I began practicing it and it has been four years since I have complained of inflammation symptoms. The trick for me was to identify that there was a problem and deal with it in a more hands-on fashion.

I made my own diet chart, changed it every few weeks and began exercising. Not only was I a few pounds lighter in no time, I was also healthy and fit in a more holistic fashion.

It took time for me to completely adapt to the anti-inflammatory diet. Now, every time I get my annual medical checkup done, the results boost my interest and reinforce my belief in the wonders of this diet.

What are the Benefits of an Anti-Inflammatory Diet?

- It helps cure mild inflammation and reduce pain and suffering.
- There are a lot of options to choose from, which makes the diet pretty flexible to follow.
- Unlike other diets, this is not a diet that leaves you hungry or staving. Instead, it provides fullness, as it requires consumption of 2000 to 3000 calories per day. The fruits and vegetables insure optimum fiber levels in the diet, which is an add-on.
- The anti-inflammatory diet has been proven to provide cardiovascular benefits. It also keeps diabetes in check by ensuring controlled sugar consumption.

- There are no additional health hazards or any side-effects to this diet.

Does it help?

It is perfectly natural to have certain apprehension, especially after reading a lot about the benefits of something. An anti-inflammatory diet is no different. In fact, it does involve a lifestyle change, which can be difficult to follow at the beginning. To answer the above question technically, I can say that it is one diet that is still undergoing much extensive research; therefore, to answer in absolutes will be too farfetched a thing to do. However, until today, the diet has only resulted in better health prospects for people who have actually made an effort to switch over to it.

Chronic disease has seen a sharp decline in people who are now following the anti-inflammatory diet. The reason for it is very obvious; the diet ensures three very important things - healthy eating, optimum weight and a physically fit body.

You have nothing to lose so why not try it and see the results for yourself!

Chapter 2: The Reasons Why You Need an Anti-Inflammatory Diet

If you are having chronic inflammation, it can be the cause of any other chronic diseases that you may have. If you manage to keep inflammation in check, you can rest assured that you have raised your guard against a number of age-related diseases and have also promoted your overall well-being. Now, since food is what we survive on, the best way to control inflammation would be to turn your regular food intake into a remedy, yet without compromising variety and taste, and moreover, without any side effects.

In cases of chronic inflammation, the body's immunity becomes responsible for fighting harmful germs such as bacteria and viruses. The immune system continuously releases chemicals that can typically be deemed responsible for warding off viruses and bacteria, but may end up becoming the cause for inflammation. Also, due to the kind of life we lead, with our chronic lack of physical activity and ever-mounting stress, chronic inflammation can occur even without the presence of external factors. An anti-inflammatory diet can help to reduce the levels of certain indicators of inflammation, such as a substance called C- reactive protein.

If you look at the daily diet of Americans today, it contains multiple food items that are saturated with omega-6 fatty acids, because of the abundance of processed foods in their diet and the lack of items that contain omega-3 fatty acids, which are good for health. Due to a poor diet, this balance between the fatty acids is upset. This is when inflammation can set in and only the right food intake, with anti-inflammatory properties, can set it right again.

In most instances of swelling, the accompanying redness occurs when there is an infection in the body. This inflammation can become the cause of serious conditions, such as cancer, heart disease, and Alzheimer's. Other factors, such as stress, physical activity, environmental toxins and diet also contribute to inflammation. The food items in your diet can either cause or combat systematic inflammation.

A well planned anti-inflammatory diet can boost both your physical and mental state and leave you energized. At the same time, it can reduce the possibility of ailments related to age, with its correct combination of fiber-rich vegetables and fruits, regulated amounts of animal protein, healthy fats, and an abundance of water. In addition, phytochemicals, which are the chemicals that exist in plant-derived food items, are also able to significantly help in reducing inflammation.

Chapter 3: What Can an Anti-Inflammatory Diet Help Treat?

Here is a list of ailments that can benefit from an anti-inflammatory diet:

Obesity
There are two facts that have been accepted widely:

1. Obesity contributes to the occurrence of inflammation and other related ailments.

2. Inflammation itself leads to an increase in the possible chances of obesity.

So whether or not the reverse of the first fact is true - that reducing weight will reduce inflammation - the second fact is enough to establish a link between an anti-inflammatory diet and weight loss. An anti-inflammatory diet, particularly one based on the Mediterranean diet, will help to keep obesity in check.

Benefits to the Cardiovascular System

The good news is that inflammation is not the main cause of cardiovascular disease; however, the concerning part is that it is more prevalent among patients suffering from heart problems. There is a definite link that connects heart disease and high concentrations of C-reactive protein (called CRP). This protein type in the the blood is an indication of inflammation.

A study has shown that this means of assessing heart risk is as efficient as the measurement of cholesterol that is used for the same purpose. The anti-inflammatory diet, because of being fiber-rich, has been shown to reduce CRP levels. Apart from lowering the risk for heart ailments, an anti-inflammatory diet also decreases "bad" LDL cholesterol and blood pressure.

Prevention and Control of Diabetes

An anti-inflammatory diet is good for both the prevention and control of diabetes. An anti-inflammatory diet helps in preventing diabetes in a number of ways. First of all, being overweight has been seen as the leading factor causing type 2 diabetes. By keeping your weight in check with an anti-inflammatory diet, you can keep the chances of diabetes at bay. In addition to that, an anti-inflammatory diet can also ward off or even reverse metabolic syndrome, which is also a cause behind heart disease and type 2 diabetes.

An anti-inflammatory diet is (or can be) mainly vegetarian, which can help in the prevention and management of diabetes. It includes the consumption of green vegetables, beans, sweet potatoes, citrus fruit, berries, etc. There are no rigid plans for meals and no pre-packaged items in the meal, so you can be sure that nothing you eat will disagree with your body, unless you are allergic to specific items.

Other Ailments That Can Be Prevented

As stated earlier, inflammation is not just a problem in itself. It can also be linked to a number of health problems, ranging from those that are lower on the danger scale to some high-risk diseases. Since nutrition and diet plans directly have an impact on the condition of inflammation in the body, following a well-designed anti-inflammatory diet plan can greatly reduce the risk (or even prevent) conditions such as allergies, cancer, asthma, Alzheimer's disease, inflammatory bowel disease (two of the most popular types being Crohn's disease and ulcerative colitis), irritable bowel syndrome and stroke.

People generally hold the opinion that any disease name that has an "itis" at the end of it involves inflammation, with common examples to support this belief being diseases such as arthritis and appendicitis. However, inflammation is much more common than that. Even the sneaky illnesses without an "itis" at the end of its name, such as certain cancers, cardiovascular disease, and even Alzheimer's disease, may actually have been triggered at least partly by inflammation. Thus, an anti-inflammatory diet is the key to correcting several health problems and diseases.

The anti-inflammatory diet is not about eating items with medicinal value; rather, it is about following a disciplined diet plan that is designed to reduce chronic cases of inflammation, a key factor in simultaneously keeping tabs on a host of other health problems and a number of diseases.

Chapter 4: In addition to an anti-inflammatory diet, you also need . . .

Lifestyle changes have the potential of dealing with the problem of inflammation in the most natural manner, which is perhaps beneficial also. Diet, as we all know, forms a major part of any lifestyle changes we might be planning to bring about. Therefore, before switching over completely to an anti-inflammatory diet, it is an absolute must to have your facts in place.

Diet Control

The focus should be on eating a healthy balanced diet. This involves maintaining a distance from pro-inflammation food products. These include fried food, processed sugar, refined carbohydrates, artificial sweeteners, trans fats and the like, which will be covered further in this book. At the same time, you must include omega-3 fats such as krill or olive oil in your diet. Omega-3 is present in fish or fish supplements and nuts such as walnuts.

Weight needs to be maintained at an optimum level at all costs. This is not directly related to an anti-inflammatory diet, nor is the diet a means to reduce weight if you're not playing sports, exercising and planning your meals properly; however, keeping your weight in check can do wonders. You need to consume as many calories as required for the daily functioning of your body. A healthy weight also keeps inflammation and pain in check.

Exercise

The next important thing that one needs to focus on is the exercise part. It is really crucial, since maintaining an optimum weight is an absolute necessity due to the fact that obesity may give rise to a plethora of problems. Exercise keeps the cholesterol levels in check and is a great way to ensure lower inflammation. In fact, one could consider taking up a hobby such as dancing or swimming, which is a great means of keeping in shape and provides entertainment and recreation at the same time. Most importantly, remember the golden rule - "what works for others might not work for you." The point is to stick to what works best for you and patiently wait for the results.

Vitamin D

An anti-inflammatory diet requires optimum insulin levels in the diet. Vitamin D levels have to be maintained; the best source for the same is proper exposure to sunlight. Vitamin D level testing should be done on a regular basis.

Give up Smoking

Smoking is another issue that needs to be tackled. It has adverse effects on health that are known to everyone. Besides, it hardens the arteries and leads to higher and unwanted levels of inflammation. For this reason, you should seriously consider giving up smoking.

Relieve Stress

Another important thing that has almost become a cliché is to stay away from stress and negative emotions. They do nothing for you other than multiplying your existing problems. This is something that is not related to our diet, but still forms a major part of all the things we need to do to keep inflammation in check. A proper diet and low levels of stress can do wonders towards building a healthy body and a sound mind. Emotional challenges need to be dealt with. Meditation can be of great help to provide inner peace and solace. If you don't know how to handle stress, I recommend that you read these two books:

-> Meditation: Beginner's Guide:

http://www.amazon.com/dp/B00KQRU9BC/

-> Stress Management with NLP:

http://www.amazon.com/dp/B00JGVZ8L0/

Chapter 5: What basically constitutes an anti-inflammatory diet?

Foods to include

Fruits and vegetables are a must have. In addition, you should consume more wholesome grains. Lean protein sources and spices, such as ginger and garlic are helpful when it comes to fighting inflammation. Drink a good quantity of water and also include berries, turmeric, beetroot, asparagus, flax seeds and avocados in your diet. In addition to the above suggested food items, I would strongly recommend the inclusion of herbs like Boswellia, camomile, bromelain, Resveratrol, melissa, primrose, borage oils and rosemary.

Dark chocolate

Unlike other sweets, dark chocolates (with a minimum cocoa content of 70%, although I recommend that you go for 90%) are ideal to keep inflammation at bay. Adding them to your diet (in moderation - they should be at the very top of your food pyramid) will help you to maintain your inclination toward eating it and at the same time ensure that you will not eat anything that can cause more harm than good.

Fatty Fish

Tuna, sardines and salmon are a few oily fish containing omega-3 fatty acids, which help in reducing inflammation. But these fish must be cooked several times a week in a healthy manner, i.e. baked or broiled, as opposed to fried or salted.

Soy

Soy contains flavones, an estrogen-like compound, which may help reduce inflammation in women. You can have soy milk, tofu and boiled soy beans.

Tomatoes

Tomatoes contain lycopene, which reduces inflammation in the body, especially the lungs. However, this depends on your symptoms and your diet. What maybe be beneficial for one person may be harmful for another and this rule applies especially to tomatoes. You should observe your reactions after consumption of tomatoes and you should stop eating them if you find your symptoms are worsening – the nightshade family of plants, to which tomatoes belong (that also include "regular" potatoes, peppers, eggplant, tomatillos, goji and other berries) contain a substance called solanine, which might cause pain in some people.

Although there aren't any official medical research findings proving the irritating properties of nightshade plants, some people claim that they get better after eliminating the nightshade plants from their diet, so you should observe your body carefully. If everything's okay, then you should definitely eat more tomatoes.

Beets

This red-colored vegetable contains anti-oxidants, fiber, vitamin C and betalains and thus has shown to reduce inflammation and protect against cancer and heart diseases.

Ginger and Turmeric

Turmeric helps in reducing NF kappa B, a protein that triggers inflammation by regulating the immune system. Thus, it helps in reducing inflammation. Ginger, if taken either as a supplement or a spice, has strong anti-inflammation properties.

Garlic and Onions

Garlic shuts down the pathways that lead to inflammation, much like many pain medications. Onion contains the phytonutrient quercetin and the compound allicin, which are anti-inflammatory chemicals.

Olive Oil

This basis of the Mediterranean diet is that it is heart-healthy and thus can also help in reducing inflammation. It contains the compound oleocanthal, which lessens inflammation.

Vegetables

Vegetables are the storehouse of many important phytonutrients and fibers, which help in keeping inflammation under control and also fights cancer, therefore you should include large quantities of raw as well as cooked vegetables in your planned diet. However, nightshade plants like "regular" potatoes and eggplant should be avoided because these contain large amounts of solanine, which can trigger inflammation in the body and even allergy, when used in large amounts in more sensitive people. On the other hand, you should definitely incorporate cruciferous vegetables and sweet potatoes into your diet.

Fruits

Fruits also contain phytonutrients, which aid the body in detoxifying itself, fight cancer and keep inflammation in check. Despite being sweet, fruits contain fiber, which modulates this sugar intake and hence does not result in the same threat to health as refined sugar. You should choose fresh or even frozen fruits, but avoid canned fruits. Smoothies made from frozen or fresh fruits, coconut milk, and veggies are another good way to add healthy calories.

Berries

Berries are high in antioxidants and low in calories and fats. They get their rich colour from anthocyanins, a chemical with anti-inflammatory properties. Tart cherries contain the highest anti-inflammatory properties compared to any other food. It is my recommendation that you should eat at least 1.5 cups of tart cherries or drink a glass of tart cherry juice a day.

Legumes

Legumes are an excellent source of vitamins, minerals, protein, fiber, and other important phytonutrients. Legumes, combined with grains, provide the body with its complete protein requirement.

Brown rice

Brown rice is a rich source of minerals, vitamins, fiber and protein. This gluten-free grain contains lignans, which is a type of phytonutrient. These lignans are converted into chemical substances in our intestines, which prevents cancer. Eating brown rice is also beneficial in decreasing insulin reactivity. Also, while white rice is a cause of constipation, brown rice helps to avoid it.

Some other gluten-free grains and grain substitutes

Arrowroot, amaranth, chestnut, artichoke, buckwheat, black rice, corn (that is, corn on the cob, cooked whole corn, tortillas, not corn flakes and other refined breakfast cereals that have a high glycemic index and lack nutrients), chickpea, red rice, oats, sweet potato, sesame, taro, quinoa and wild rice are some grains that you should include in your diet as much as you can.

Nuts and seeds

If you are not allergic to nuts then you might include three tablespoons of nuts to your diet, preferably unsalted and with no add-ons. They add fiber and Omega-3 fatty acids to your diet. Almonds and peanuts can also be consumed in moderate quantities, again unless you have a history of nut allergy.

Lemon water

Simply consuming a glass of water with lemon squeezed in it affords a number of health benefits. It alkalinizes your body, cleanses and detoxifies it and helps to strengthen the immune system, while simultaneously supplying nutrients like bioflavonoid and vitamin C to the body. Try to drink warm water and lemon every day.

Coconut milk

There cannot be a better substitute for dairy products than coconut milk. Medium chain triglycerides (shortened as MCTs), chemicals present in coconut milk, are easy to digest and hence they are easily combusted to give energy to the pancreas, liver and the digestive system with bare effort. The benefit lies in the MTCs, which are an anti-inflammatory and also contribute to maintaining a strong immune system. There are a number of ways in which coconut milk can be consumed: plain coconut water, coconut water and rice milk mixture, in <u>smoothies</u> and also in various recipes replacing cream, milk and other dairy products. You can also include coconut oil and unsweetened coconut meat in your diet.

Food items to avoid or limit

While there is enough said about what you must include in your diet, it is necessary to pay attention to what you should not. Although there are different food items for different people, (as we discussed earlier) simply follow the age old rule of "what works for you might not work for others." Still, there are some food items which you must avoid at all costs.

GMO

GMO stands for Genetically Modified Organisms. Consumption of these types of genetically modified food items can cause severe inflammation. This is because the body is not able to break them down, so they remain undigested, and sooner or later escape they into the blood. The immune system, on encountering such elements, goes haywire and causes inflammation.

Trans Fat

Trans fats are a big no-no. They not only cause obesity and other diseases, but also induce inflammation by damaging the cells in the lining of the blood vessels.

Sugar

Today we consume sugar in almost everything, but our body is not meant to break down so much sugar. A lot of sugar leads to immunity messengers known as cytokines, which causes inflammation. You should definitely avoid it and use maple syrup or honey as an alternative.

Cheeseburgers (and any other fast-food)

Fast-foods contain saturated fats, which has a compound known as arachidonic acid that naturally creates inflammation, but some saturated fats are necessary for the body, so consume this in moderation.

Alcohol and Coffee

Ah! Alcohol and coffee. The assumed cause of all evils can lead to inflammation if consumed in large quantities, as it would enable bacteria to pass easily through your intestines, causing irritation and inflammation. Instead, you can drink red grape wine (the perfect amount would be no more than 1 glass a day) and/or green tea.

Omega-6 Fatty Acids

Remember how Omega-3 fatty acids reduced inflammation? Well, on the contrary Omega-6 fatty acids can increase the risk of inflammation. Your body can't produce them and so they need to be regularly provided to keep your organs functioning properly - they constitute a component of cell membranes, play an important role in the immune system and protect us from the development of inflammatory conditions, **BUT** they should be consumed in moderation. They are found in large amounts in vegetable oils (coconut, sunflower, corn, grape seed, peanut, sesame oil, soy and margarines produced from them) and heavy seeds. You should also remember that you should consume these oils in their raw form (drizzling on your salads, etc.), and not use them for frying. When it comes to frying, I recommend that you stick to olive oil and grape seed oil.

Eggs, meats

During the process of digestion of animal proteins, the body creates acids and other by-products that can potentially be toxic and inflammatory. White meat (which includes fish and poultry), poses a lower danger to health than varieties of red meats, so completely avoid red meats such as pork and beef in your diet. On the other hand, cold-water fish like salmon contains Omega-3 fatty acids, which are anti-inflammatory. You can include lean poultry and fish in your diet, but make sure it is in moderation, that is to say, not more than two servings per day. Limit your consumption of eggs to one serving on alternate days, or consume egg whites with the yolks removed - they contain arachidonic acid.

Wheat and other grains containing gluten

Gluten-containing grains, barley and wheat contain proteins which lead to excessive production of immunoglobulin. It can be responsible for provoking an inflammatory reaction. They should be consumed rarely. Let us also look at white bread, the most common of all food items in our daily lives. The reason for placing white bread on this list is that it easily breaks down into sugar, which in turn leads to inflammation.

Dairy products

Dairy products can provoke an inflammatory reaction in the body because they contain proteins responsible for the production of immunoglobulin, which is a direct cause of inflammation. So you should limit the consumption of milk from goats and cows, and all other products derived from them, such as cheese - especially the "full fat" products! If your body can tolerate organic cultured dairy products like kefir, natural yogurt, etc., then a moderate quantity of these can be included in your diet plan.

Miscellaneous

Other food items to be avoided in an anti-inflammatory diet are fried foods, particular food items that you are allergic to (with allergic foods being a cause of inflammation), potatoes, yams, food additives like colors, preservatives, artificial flavors, sweeteners and hydrogenated (trans) fats, as well as sugary items.

Chapter 6: The healthiest ways to cook anti-inflammatory foods

The manner of cooking foods also gains a lot of importance when it comes to following a proper anti-inflammatory diet.

Fried foods are a big no because they give rise to a lot of problems. Instead, boiling and steaming food is preferred over the traditional method of frying. Although frying is said to accentuate the flavour of the food, it poses a threat to one's health in the long run. It adds a lot more calories, fats and cholesterol, which are not beneficial for the body.

On the other hand, boiling, roasting and steaming are healthier options, though you might dislike the taste initially. Over time, one develops a taste for these foods and in fact, variations in the diet can help you to develop a liking for certain foods prepared using these methods, so do not worry.

Flaxseed oil and olive oil can be mixed with foods we eat, such as cottage cheese or pasta, and their nutty taste actually mingles with these food items and provides a good taste and texture. Flaxseed oil can be sprinkled on cereals or fruits and can thus be easily incorporated in the diet. From breakfast to snacks to main courses to dessert, try supplementing everything with something healthy and tasty. Trust me, once you begin, you will find a plethora of options and you will never want to go back.

The most important aspect of an anti-inflammatory diet is that it requires not only the right ingredients, but also the appropriate and correct means of cooking them. As a matter of fact, one can lose a lot of nutritional value from food simply by cooking it in an inappropriate manner. We tend to do this pretty often, sometimes due to prioritizing taste over health.

Best Cooking Methods

Let us have a close look at the suggested means of cooking that one needs to adopt in order to follow a proper anti-inflammatory diet:

- Baking: This is a highly accepted mode of cooking. What is required is simply to place the food on a ceramic baking dish with ample space on the sides to allow for the circulation of hot air. Cooking veggies or meat on the dish in a set up like this makes room for moisture to seep in. This retains the nutrient content, enhances flavours and keeps the natural juices of the food intact.

- Steaming: One of the most common means of cooking food, steaming, can be done easily in a number of ways. A bamboo steamer or a rice steamer are pretty popular modes of cooking that employ steaming. In fact, one can create his/her own steamer by using a covered pot with a slotted insert and can use this to cook a variety of food according to one's taste. Care must be taken to ensure that the food is not overcooked, especially veggies, meat and fish. At the same time, before placing the food on a steamer, marinate it properly with appropriate herbs and add spices like ginger and turmeric to infuse a rich flavour into the food.

- Poaching: Poaching is one of the simplest and least troublesome means of cooking and requires no extra fats. It just requires water or stock, thereby cutting down on additional fats. Bring the poaching liquid to a boiling point and add the vegetables, seafood and meat to it. Lower the heat and simmer for a while. The poaching liquid can serve other purposes after taking out the cooked veggies or meat. It could be used as a base for soup, which enhances the taste and is extremely healthy.

- Stir-frying: An excellent substitute for normal frying, stir-frying is used to cook vegetables in a smaller quantity of oil at a high temperature. The cooking time is less, thus a little oil seeps inside the food, and therefore it retains the natural flavour and nutritional qualities and also offers a tasty meal.

- Grilling and broiling: These are means best suited for vegetables and fish. This method does not work very well for meats, as prolonged exposure to high temperature raises the risk of cancer by increasing the heterocyclic amine content in food.

- Microwaving of food is also a method that can be used, especially for warming purposes, but prolonged exposure of food to heat should be avoided as it poses hazards in the long run.

- Cooking with ice: This means can preserve flavours and ingredients, but also rehydrate food and change textures. However, it works best for herbs.

The use of Omega-6 polyunsaturated plant oils in cooking should be reduced. Instead, olive oil should be used for all such purposes. Foods cooked at extremely high temperatures should be avoided. These create pro-inflammatory compounds, which are again hazardous. Meats should be stir-fried, sautéed and slow cooked, while veggies should be boiled and steamed.

Steaming is quick and it preserves nutrients. The vegetables and meat should be cut into an appropriate size to facilitate steaming and stir-frying. One of the most important things that we tend to overlook includes the smoking of oils that should be avoided at all costs. For example, extra virgin oil should not be exposed to a temperature above 325 F, but this kind of temperature is rather difficult to get using ordinary home cooking methods.

A key piece of advice is in maintaining the correct attitude while cooking. A hurried meal or a meal prepared while in a stressed state will never turn out to be perfect. In fact, it will lead to stressful flavours. Cooking is an art of self-reflection and how we cook is as important as what we eat. It deserves proper attention, patience and time.

Chapter 7: Recipes and daily diet plan

Okay, so are you all geared up to take on an anti-inflammatory diet? Great, but before you begin let me caution you into setting up a support system that can give you strength when you feel like giving it up altogether. There will be numerous instances of resistance and so do not be afraid, it will be just fine! You will sail through the tough times smoothly. To make sure that this diet regimen does not turn out to be a sacrificial exercise, try and explore fun recipes, and try to devise an even better means of preparing them. Most importantly, enjoy, chill out and relax!

An anti-inflammatory diet focuses on curtailing the excessive calorie intake and at the same time ensures you begin to like the diet. To begin with, let us have a look at the recipe of c**elery soup.** It is healthy, tasty and beneficial.

Celery Soup

Serves: 4

Ingredients:

- 1 tbsp. olive oil
- Bunch of chopped celery
- 4 green onions, chopped
- 1 russet potato of medium size
- 1 medium sized leek with white and light green parts, finely chopped
- 4 cups of water with 0.5 teaspoon of salt or 4 cups of low sodium chicken broth
- chopped fresh parsley and fat-free yogurt or coconut milk/cream

Directions:

1. Heat the oil on medium heat in a stockpot and add all the veggies along with celery.
2. Stir occasionally until the vegetables get tender (at least 8-10 minutes).
3. Now add the potato along with the water or the chicken broth.
4. Boil further. Let the soup cook for about 8-10 minutes until the potato becomes tender.
5. Remove from heat and let it cool for another 10 minutes.
6. Let the soup cool down, pour into the blender and mix with the yogurt until you get a smooth puree.
7. Keep the soup in the refrigerator.
8. This soup is best served chilled, sprinkled with parsley.

Orange Salmon Salad

Serves: 2

Ingredients:

- 2 cups of green lettuce, preferably dark coloured
- ¼ cups of grated carrot and red onion
- 1 teaspoon olive oil
- vinegar to taste
- Seasoning of choice – I like it with basil and oregano or herbs de Provence.
- ½ cup soft goat cheese and salmon (you can also replace the salmon with another type of fish of your choice.)

Directions:

1. In a large bowl, place the lettuce, onion and carrot and mix well.
2. Now add the olive oil, vinegar and seasonings.
3. Drizzle the seasonings and the salad well and put them over the cheese and salmon.
4. This can be served with whole wheat bread or seedless grapes.
5. Also, any calorie free drink or tea can be served as a beverage alongside this fabulous salad.

White Bean and Chicken Chili Blanca

Serves: 4

Ingredients:

- 1.1 lbs. (about 500 g) 2 boneless and skinless chicken breasts, cut into cubes
- extra virgin olive oil
- 2 onions and 4 cloves of garlic, diced
- 1 cup white or great northern beans, drained and rinsed
- corn kernels (preferably fresh), half cup
- chopped chilli, to taste
- ¼ teaspoon ground cumin
- ½ teaspoon chili powder
- pepper, to taste
- 3 cups water
- 100% natural low fat parmesan cheese – go for high quality Parmesan
- Cilantro chopped.

The quantity of these ingredients depends upon the number of people it is made for and the time is approximately 20 minutes.

Directions:

1. To begin with, season the chicken with salt and pepper.
2. Add oil to a pan and heat it. Then add the chicken pieces and cook for 3-4 minutes.
3. Now, lower the heat and add garlic and onion to the chicken and fry until the onion softens.

4. Add the rest of the ingredients.
5. Add water and bring it to a boil.
6. After this, leave it uncovered and let it simmer for a while.
7. Garnish each serving with cheese and cilantro.

Barley Salad

Serves: 3

Ingredients:

- 1-1.5 cups of uncooked barley
- ½ cup fresh corn kernels
- 2 diced and seeded plum tomatoes
- 1 onion, chopped
- parsley to taste
- Kalamata olives
- freshly squeezed lemon juice
- olive oil
- salt
- black pepper
- garlic, 2 cloves
- 100% natural low fat crumbled cheese

The quantity of veggies can vary from a cup to two. Salt to taste and oils and juices to 2-3 tablespoon.

Directions:

1. Cook the barley first in lightly salted water, following the instructions on the package.
2. Drain, rinse and cool completely.
3. Combine the barley with corn kernels and the other ingredients.
4. Add the juice and other ingredients.
5. Toss to coat and sprinkle with cheese.

Tuscan White Bean Stew

Serves: 5

Ingredients:

To make the croutons, you will need-

- 1 tablespoon extra-virgin olive oil
- 2 garlic cloves, cut into smaller parts
- 8 sliced brown bread cut into cubes
- 2 cups white beans dried and rinsed
- 6 cups water
- salt to taste
- 1 bay leaf
- 2 tablespoon olive oil
- 1 yellow onion, chopped and peeled
- 3 carrots, peeled and cut into cubes
- 6 garlic cloves, chopped finely
- 1 tablespoon fresh rosemary

- black pepper to taste
- 1-1.5 cups of natural vegetable stock or broth

Directions:

1. Heat the oil in a large frying pan.
2. Add 2 garlic cloves cut into small pieces and sauté for a minute.
3. Remove from heat and let the garlic flavour totally sink into the oil for 10 minutes.
4. Discard the garlic pieces and put the pan back on the heat.
5. Add the brown bread cubes and sauté until light brown. Remove and set aside.
6. In a soup pot, combine bay leaf, water, salt and beans.
7. Bring to a boil and cook for about an hour until the beans become tender and soft.
8. Drain the beans and reserve half of the cooking liquid.
9. Discard the bay leaves. Place the beans into a large pot.
10. Now use the reserved liquid and half of the cooked beans.
11. Prepare them into a paste.
12. In the cooking pot, again heat olive oil.
13. Add onion and carrot and sauté till crisp.
14. Add chopped garlic and add the rest of the spices.
15. Add bean mixture and the stock.
16. Bring to a boil and simmer until the stew is heated. Ideally, this will take about 5 minutes.
17. Serve as desired, garnished with rosemary sprig.

Asian Vegetable Salad

Serves: 2

Ingredients:

- rice vinegar
- honey, 2 teaspoons
- garlic and chilli olive oil
- gluten-free soy sauce (low sodium)
- 1+1 teaspoon organic grass-feed butter
- slivered almond
- sunflower seeds
- 1 cup soy noodles, cooked
- ½ cup Chinese cabbage
- 1 green onion, sliced
- ½ cup carrots, cut into small cubes

Directions:

1. Combine the first five ingredients and bring to a boil.
2. Now spoon the mixture into a bowl and let it chill.
3. Add butter to a non-stick pan and heat it on medium heat.
4. Add almonds, sunflower kernels and noodles.
5. Cook for 3 minutes. Toss lightly.
6. Combine both the mixtures together and mix well.
7. Let stand for 15 minutes then add the remaining vegetables.
8. You can sprinkle it with few drops of sesame oil before serving.

Indian Spiced Carrot Soup with Ginger

Serves: 2

Ingredients:

- a handful coriander and mustard seeds
- olive oil
- 1 teaspoon curry powder,
- 2 chopped onions
- Part of fresh ginger root, peeled and minced
- 2 chopped carrots
- Peel of 1 lime, grated
- 1 ½ cup 100% natural chicken or vegetable broth
- freshly squeezed lime juice
- 3 tbsp. coconut milk

Directions:

1. Grind together coriander and mustard seed to a fine powder.
2. Heat oil in a pan over medium heat and add ground seeds and curry powder.
3. Add ginger and other ingredients.
4. Sprinkle with salt and pepper and sauté till onions soften.
5. Now add the broth and bring it to a boil.
6. Wait until the carrots are tender and then cool them.
7. Working in batches, puree in blender until smooth.
8. Return soup to pot. If you find it too thick, add more broth.
9. Stir in lime juice and add salt and pepper.
10. Ladle the soup into bowls and serve garnished with coconut milk.

One Week Diet Plan

In addition to the above, you could also try a seven day diet plan that would work wonders. Try it for four weeks and observe your body.

Day 1
- **Breakfast**: Spinach and Mushroom Frittata

Serves: 2-3
Ingredients:

- 6 eggs
- 1 small onion, chopped finely or cut into small cubes (you can also use small leek)
- 8.8 oz. (250 grams) boletus or champignons – rinsed, drained and cut in quarters
- 4.2 oz. (120 g) fresh spinach leaves (try not to buy frozen spinach if possible) , rinsed, drained, chopped coarsely
- 1 clove grated garlic
- 2 tbsp. grated natural Parmesan cheese (go for a good quality Parmesan)
- 3 tbsp. olive oil
- salt, black pepper

Directions:

1. Fry the onion and mushrooms in a pan with a thick bottom, stirring from time to time.
2. Add spinach and garlic, fry for 2 minutes, then reduce the heat.
3. Beat the eggs and season them with salt and pepper.
4. Pour the eggs, mushrooms, onion and garlic into a casserole dish slightly smeared with olive oil or grass-fed butter.
5. Preheat oven to 360 F (180 C), then bake for about 20 minutes until the mixture becomes dense and slightly browned.
6. Cut your frittata in halves, serve with rice waffles or fresh whole grain bread.

- **Lunch**: Pumpkins served with ginger have excellent anti-inflammatory properties that you don't want to miss. Just add green salad and there you go!

Serves: 2

Ingredients:

- ½ small pumpkin (about 10 inch/25 cm in diameter) peeled, cut into 1 inch (~2 cm) cubes
- 2 tbsp. organic honey
- 2 teaspoons freshly squeezed lemon juice
- ½ teaspoon peeled and freshly grated ginger
- 4 tbsp. fresh Greek yoghurt
- 3 tbsp. sliced walnuts roasted in a skillet
- freshly ground black pepper

Directions:

1. Simmer pumpkin in the saucepan with ½ cup water for about 10 minutes until tender.
2. Add honey, lemon juice, ginger, heat for a while.
3. Put pumpkin into the bowls. Evaporate the sauce if it's too thin.
4. Mix the sauce with yogurt and nuts, then season with pepper and add to the bowls.

The pumpkin seeds contain healthy oil (about 40%) along with 0.7% minerals and more than 1% fiber. There are also proteins, sugars, enzymes, resins, vitamin A, B9 and B15. Pumpkin seeds are high in zinc and lecithin. They also contain other minerals such as potassium, calcium, phosphorus, magnesium, which all increase metabolism and support your brain.

- **Dinner**: Sweet Potato and Black Bean Burger with Lime Dip!

Serves: 3

Ingredients:

- 1 cup dry black beans
- 1 yellow onion, peeled and cut into cubes
- ½ red onion, peeled and cut into cubes
- 2 cloves garlic, finely sliced
- 1 tbsp. olive oil
- 1 cup oat flakes
- 1 fresh red chili pepper

- 2 teaspoons roasted pepper
- ½ teaspoon ground coriander
- 1 teaspoon ground cumin
- handful of freshly chopped coriander
- salt
- 1 sweet potato, peeled and boiled in slightly salted water with few drops of olive oil

Directions:

1. Soak the beans overnight, then cook in unsalted water until tender.
2. Heat the olive oil in a saucepan, add onion and garlic, fry until browned.
3. Soak the oat flakes in 1/3 cup water and cook until all the water is absorbed and the flakes are tender.
4. Combine the cooled cooked beans with browned vegetables and spices. Put everything into the food processor/blender and mix for just a few seconds, but do not over-blend the mixture.
5. Add cooked oats and fresh coriander, mix with a spoon and let stand in a cool place for 30 minutes.
6. Once the mixture is cooled properly, form burgers and fry in olive oil until both sides are golden brown.
7. Put the burgers on a baking tray lined with baking paper. Preheat oven to 360 F (180 C) and bake for about 15 minutes.
8. Serve the burgers with the lime dip and boiled sweet potato. You can also add a tiny pinch of cayenne pepper (chili powder).

Lime dip:

Ingredients:

- 3 tbsp canola-based mayonnaise
- 2 tbsp Greek yoghurt
- Juice and grated peel of ¼ lime
- one pinch turmeric
- 2 pinches Cayenne pepper
- a pinch of salt
- 1/3 tsp spicy chili sauce (or more, to taste)

Directions:

1. Mix yogurt with cayenne pepper, chili sauce and a pinch of salt.
2. After one minute, add lemon and grated peel of ¼ lime.
3. Wait for another moment and add turmeric.
4. Blend everything thoroughly using a spoon.

Day 2

- **Breakfast**: Smoothies are a nice option to begin your day with. Go with the fruit of your choice and Greek yogurt. You can also make this fresh and delicious smoothie:

Kiwi and Pineapple Smoothie

Serves: 2

Ingredients:

- 2 kiwis, peeled
- 10 oz. (300 ml) 100% natural pineapple juice
- 2 bananas, peeled and cut into smaller parts

Directions:

1. Put peeled kiwi into the blender and pour in cold pineapple juice.
2. Add bananas.
3. Blend everything until smooth. Pour into cups and enjoy!

The smoothie is a vitamin bomb.

Kiwi is a cumulative dose of vitamin C and E, an excellent fruit, which enhances the immune system, reducing the time it takes to treat infection, and above all, prevents depression. Pineapple has both potent anti-inflammatory and digestive properties and is also useful in times of high stress. I would heartily recommend this fruit - as it is just perfect for every state of mind.

Or you can try this one:

Ingredients:

Serves: 2

- 5.3 oz. (about 0.6 cups,150g) kale, thoroughly rinsed and drained
- 2 bananas, peeled
- 27 oz. (800 ml) fresh 100% natural orange juice
- 2 tbsp. honey
- thumb-sized fresh ginger root, peeled and finely grated
- few tbsp. lemon juice (to taste)

Directions:

1. Put ginger, kale and bananas into a blender/food processor and shred for one minute.
2. Add orange juice, honey and lemon juice and blend for minute or two until smooth.
3. Pour into cups and enjoy!

You can also find lots of great, healthy smoothie ideas in this book of mine: http://www.amazon.com/dp/B00J8ZHMIQ/

- **Lunch**: Go with kippers' salad, as it is a source of Omega-3 fatty acids. Combine this with whole wheat bread for a wholesome meal.

Serves: 2

Ingredients:

- 4 fillets of herring in oil – cut into cubes
- 2 sweet potatoes - rinsed, cooked in slightly salted water, peeled and cut into cubes
- 2 pickles – cut into cubes
- 4 tbsp. Greek yoghurt
- a pinch of chili powder to taste
- ½ red onion
- a bunch of parsley, finely sliced
- salt and freshly ground black pepper to taste
- 10-15 black olives

Directions:

Thoroughly mix all the salad ingredients in a bowl. Serve chilled.

- **<u>Dinner</u>**: You can stick to a big bowl of chilli:

Ingredients:

- 1.1 lbs. (500 grams) organic lamb, cut against the grain and into cubes
- 2 red bell peppers, sliced, with removed core
- 15 oz. red boiled beans (try not to use canned beans if possible)

- 2 red onions, minced
- 1 clove garlic, minced
- 2 chili peppers (or less if you don't like it too spicy), with removed seeds, chopped finely
- 2 tbsp. natural tomato paste (or you can also blend one small tomato in a blender/food processor with a pinch of Italian seasoning)
- 15 oz. skinned tomatoes (peeled using boiled water)
- 2-3 tbsp olive oil
- salt, paprika, black pepper to taste
- basil and oregano – preferably fresh

Directions:

1. Fry the lamb, garlic and onion in the preheated olive oil until the meat and veggies are slightly brown.
2. Add tomato paste and 3/4 cup water; season with salt and pepper, stir thoroughly and then simmer for 40 minutes.
3. Add red bell peppers and chili peppers and simmer for another 15 minutes over low heat, stirring occasionally.
4. Add red beans and simmer for another 5 minutes. Toward the end of the cooking time, sprinkle with fresh basil and oregano and season with salt and black pepper to taste. Serve with whole wheat bread. Enjoy!

Day 3

<u>Breakfast:</u> Gingerbread oatmeal. This is an easy recipe, which is both healthy and nutritious.

Serves: 3
Ingredients:

- 1 cup oats
- 1 handful cranberries
- ginger
- cinnamon
- nutmeg
- 2 cups water
- ¼ cup flaxseeds
- 1 cup molasses

Directions:

1. In a small saucepan add water, oats, cranberries, ginger, cinnamon and nutmeg.
2. Bring it to boil and simmer for about 5 minutes, until the oats absorb the water.
3. Now add flaxseed to the above and let it sit for some time.
4. While serving, pair it up with molasses.

- **Lunch**: Roasted chicken wrap

Serves: 2-3
Ingredients:

- 2 small chicken breasts - about 0.8 lbs. (400 g) – rinsed, drained
- herbal pepper
- lemon pepper
- thyme
- oregano
- sweet paprika powder
- 1 carrot, cut into long strips
- ½ red bell pepper, cut into long strips
- a few leaves of *Lollo Rossa* lettuce
- 1 fresh cucumber, cut into long strips
- 1 tbsp. chopped parsley
- 1 tbsp. grape seed oil
- 1 clove garlic, finely chopped

Sauce:
- 3 tbsp. Greek yoghurt
- 4 tbsp. canola-based mayonnaise
- 2 cloves garlic, grated
- freshly squeezed lemon juice – to taste
- salt and pepper to taste

Additionally:
4 gluten-free tortilla wraps
1. **Prepare the chicken:** Preheat the oven to 450 F (230 C).
2. Season the chicken with salt, lemon and herbal pepper, sweet paprika powder, thyme and oregano. Drizzle with olive oil.

3. Put the chicken in a shallow casserole dish or arrange on a heat-resistant tray lined with baking paper, smeared with olive oil (unless it's Teflon or a similar dish with a nonstick coating) and leave uncovered for 5 minutes.
4. Lower the temperature to 430 F (220 C) and roast for 10 minutes. Flip the breasts upside down at least once during the roasting.
5. **Prepare the vegetables:** Preheat the olive oil in the saucepan, add garlic, and stir fry for a moment, then add carrot and red bell pepper.
6. Fry for a moment, stirring occasionally, so that vegetables remain slightly hard (al dente), not entirely tender.
7. Season with salt and pepper, and add the chicken breast to heat it up.
8. Remove from the heat, add chopped parsley and stir.
9. **Prepare the sauce**: Mix mayonnaise with yogurt, add grated garlic, season with lemon juice, salt and freshly ground black pepper.
10. Rinse and dry the lettuce.
11. Heat tortilla wraps in a preheated skillet (no oil) on both sides, about 30 seconds each, or according to the directions on the package.
12. Smear the warm wraps with sauce, arrange lettuce leaves, cucumber and diced chicken with vegetables. You can also sprinkle it with few drops of olive oil.
13. Roll the wraps. In case you are not sure how to do it or you are looking for new ideas, you can follow this link:

http://www.wikihow.com/Fold-a-Tortilla

14. Serve the tortillas immediately. Enjoy!

- **Dinner**: Who said eggs are just for breakfast? Try poached eggs with curried vegetables:

Serves: 3
Ingredients

- 3 eggs
- 1 cup mushrooms
- 2 onions
- 1 garlic
- 2 small zucchinis (courgettes)
- 1 teaspoon yellow curry powder
- olive oil
- 1 cup chickpeas
- 1 red bell pepper
- vinegar

Directions:

1. Sauté onions and garlic in a non-stick pan and add the yellow curry powder until the aroma emerges.
2. Add mushrooms and cook them until tender, stopping once they give out water.

3. Add the zucchinis, red pepper, vinegar and water and bring them to a boil. This should take approximately 15-20 minutes.
4. Meanwhile, in a different pan, add water to a depth of at least 3 inches in order to soak the eggs well.
5. Add vinegar and one by one add the eggs.
6. Simmer the eggs and carefully remove them with a slotted spoon.
7. Mix the veggies and eggs and the dinner is ready for you to enjoy!

Day 4

- **Breakfast:** All-natural turkey sausage and whole bread drizzled with chilli-garlic olive oil.

- **Lunch:** Fruit salad with berries, kiwis and citrus - 1 cups berries, one kiwi, one lemon or lime, 2 tbsp. desiccated coconut or roasted pumpkin seeds. You should also add natural honey to taste (about 2 tbsp.) and two tbsp. natural Tahini (sesame paste) - it's sooo delicious!

- **Dinner:** Oven baked cod. Served with roasted butternut squash and sprinkled with turmeric:

Serves: 2-3
Ingredients:

- 2-4 (about 14 oz., 400 g) cod fillets, rinsed and drained
- 1 carrot

- ½ leek
- 1 zucchini (courgette)
- ½ red bell pepper, cut into strips
- ½ yellow pepper, cut into strips
- a piece of celery, peeled, cut into strips
- 1 medium spring onion, diced
- 2-3 sweet potatoes, cut into rounds
- 1 clove garlic, finely chopped
- 1 tiny piece of chili pepper, finely chopped
- 1 teaspoon natural fish seasoning
- few leaves basil – preferably fresh
- juice of ½ lemon
- 2 tbsp olive oil
- salt
- lemon pepper
- green parsley, finely chopped

Directions:

1. Drizzle the fish with lemon juice on both sides, smear with olive oil combined with fish seasoning. Season with salt, pepper, garlic and chili.
2. Put into the refrigerator for about 20-30 minutes in a closed container.

3. Prepare the aluminum foil. Put extra baking paper in the middle of the foil and gently smear it with olive oil.

4. Arrange the fish and vegetables (slightly seasoned with salt) on the paper. Wrap everything in aluminum foil to form a packet with the top closed, which you will then put into the casserole and bake in the oven preheated to 360 F (180 C) for about 25-30 minutes.

5. At the end, you can gently unfold the foil to slightly brown the fish.

6. Put baked fish on a platter. Fold the foil on the sides along the fish and sprinkle it with chopped parsley and basil.

7. Extras are rather redundant here, but you can have organic whole grain bread or a roasted butternut squash (peeled, seeded and cut in halves - just arrange it on a baking tray lined with baking paper, flesh side up, season with salt and pepper, drizzle with olive oil and put in the oven along with the cod) and a glass of good wine.

In between meals, you could munch on almonds and pumpkin seeds.

Day 5

- **Breakfast**: Begin the day with ginger-apple muffins served with tea or a calorie-free beverage.

Serves: 1-2
Ingredients:

- 1 large carrot, peeled and grated finely
- 1 apple, peeled and grated finely
- 3.5 oz. (100 g) wheat flour and 3.5 oz. rice flour **or** 7 oz. (200 g) of Schar flour mix C
- 2.8 oz. 100% high quality natural yoghurt
- 2 heaped tablespoons natural clarified butter + some more to grease the muffin tins
- 2 tbsp. crushed almonds/ almond flakes
- 1/3 cup honey
- 2.8 oz. (80 g) dark gluten-free chocolate, cut into smaller parts
- 1 tbsp baking soda
- 2 eggs
- 1 teaspoon cinnamon
- ½ teaspoon ground ginger
- ½ teaspoon nutmeg

Directions:

1. Melt the butter and set aside to allow it to cool. In the meantime, grease the muffin tins.
2. Preheat the oven to 320 F (160 C).
3. Beat the eggs in the bowl. Add flour, soda, and yogurt and mix thoroughly.
4. Add grated carrot and apples, nutmeg, cinnamon, ginger, molten butter, honey and chopped chocolate. Mix again thoroughly. Pour into tins - 3/4 height.
5. Sprinkle with almond flakes/crushed almonds and put in the oven for 40 minutes. Remember that you should check the oven occasionally, and you may use a long thin stick to check to see if the muffins are ready - just put the stick inside the muffin - if it's dry after you remove it, the muffins are ready! Enjoy!

- **Lunch**: You could go for chocolate pear salad (two pears, apple, 2 tbsp. maple syrup or honey, 5 cubes dark crushed chocolate, ½ handful crushed walnuts, 3 tsp sesame seeds) or any salad for that matter. Salads are healthy lunch options.

- **Dinner**: Opt for red pepper turkey pasta. Red peppers are rich in vitamin C. The recipe is simple and easy to cook.

Serves: 3

Ingredients

- 2 red bell peppers
- 2 onions
- garlic
- red wine vinegar
- 2 cups Rigatoni pasta, cooked al dente in slightly salted water with 1 teaspoon olive oil
- oregano
- olive oil
- 1 cup ground turkey

Directions:

1. The peppers should be cut in halves and the seeds should be removed carefully.
2. Cook onions, garlic and peppers in a pan along with olive oil.
3. Once cool, transfer the mixture in a blender and make a puree.
4. Add oregano to season. Now sauté turkey and simmer for 2 minutes and add to hot pasta. Serve with sauce.

Day 6

- **Breakfast:** Add quinoa to the traditional oatmeal porridge and garnish it with tart cherries. This can be a delicious and very healthy change from the regular breakfast recipe!

- **Lunch**: Delicious roasted sweet potato soup!

Serves: 2-3

Ingredients:

- 2 sweet potatoes – rinsed, unpeeled, cut into thick slices
- 1 garlic clove
- a piece of ginger root
- 1 medium shallot
- a pinch of chili rings
- sea salt, freshly ground black pepper
- 3 cups (about 24 oz., 0.7 L) natural vegetable broth
- Optionally: 1 tbsp. coconut milk cream

Directions:

1. Drizzle the sweet potato slices with olive oil and bake in the oven preheated to 390 F (200 C) until tender.
2. Remove from the oven, cool down, peel and mix in a blender.
3. Chop all the vegetables, fry in olive oil and add to the sweet potato puree.
4. Mix again until smooth.

5. Add the vegetable broth, mix again, transfer to the pot and cook for 5 minutes over low heat.

6. Season with pepper, chili and oregano.

7. I recommend that you also add one tablespoon coconut milk or coconut milk cream. The soup will be even more delicate and appetizing!

- **Dinner:** Let's prepare aromatic steamed salmon with lemon-scented zucchini!

Serves: 2

Ingredients:

- about 11 oz. (~300 g) salmon steaks, rinsed and drained

- 2 young zucchinis (courgettes), rinsed, dried, with cut out tops

- 2 carrots, rinsed, dried, peeled

- 1 tbsp grass-fed butter

- half a bunch of fresh thyme

- half a bunch of fresh basil

- freshly squeezed lemon juice

- salt

- freshly ground black pepper

- 2 yams, peeled and cooked in slightly salted water

Directions:

1. Season the salmon with salt and pepper on both sides and drizzle with lemon juice.

2. Put in the refrigerator for 30 minutes.

3. Using a vegetable peeler, cut the carrot and zucchini in thin ribbons (tagliatelle).

4. Place two cups of water in a steam cooker. Put in basil and thyme, cook for 5 minutes.

5. Arrange the salmon and vegetable tagliatelle on the perforated inset and place over boiling water. Cover and cook on steam (on low power/heat) for 10 to 15 minutes.

6. Once ready and still hot, add extra thin grass-fed butter slices or drizzle with olive oil. Serve with cooked yams.

7. If you don't have a steam cooker yet (or a pot suitable for steam cooking), you can just carefully wrap the salmon in aluminum foil, put on a baking tray and bake in the oven preheated to 300 F (~150 C) for 30 minutes.

Day 7

- **Breakfast:** Gluten-free strawberry crepes

Serves: 2

Ingredients:

- ½ cup Schar Mix C flour
- water
- 1 tsp grape seed oil or olive oil
- 1-2 cups strawberries (fresh if possible) or other berries, rinsed, dried and cut into smaller parts
- honey or maple syrup

Directions:

1. Mix the flour with oil in the bowl. Gradually add the water while vigorously stirring with a spoon until the mixture reaches a pancake batter consistency.
2. Fry in a Teflon saucepan (slightly smeared with oil) on both sides, just like regular pancakes.
3. Drizzle the pancakes with honey or maple syrup, arrange strawberries and roll wraps or fold in triangles.
4. The pancakes can be served both warm and cold. Enjoy!

- **Lunch:** Quinoa and Turkey Stuffed Peppers

Serves: 2
Ingredients:

- ½ cup quinoa
- 11 oz. (~300 g) minced turkey meat
- 1 small onion, finely chopped

- 8.8 oz. (250 g) fresh green peas, peeled
- 2 large ripe tomatoes
- salt, pepper
- olive oil
- fresh herbs: e.g. basil and oregano
- 4 large bell peppers – rinsed, drained, with tops cut off, hollowed

Garlic sauce:
- 7 oz (200 g) Greek yoghurt
- 1 clove garlic, minced
- salt, pepper

Directions:
1. Combine Greek yogurt with minced garlic, season with salt and pepper (you can also add few drops of fresh lemon juice) and put in the refrigerator.
2. Cook the ½ cup quinoa in 1 cup slightly salted water.
3. Preheat the olive oil and slightly brown the onion. Then add minced turkey and fry. Once meat starts changing color, add peas and tomatoes.
4. Simmer for about 15 minutes, stirring occasionally. Season with salt, pepper and herbs.
5. Evaporate the excess fluids, add cooked quinoa and stir thoroughly.
   Season if needed.
6. Fill the hollowed peppers with the stuffing and arrange in a casserole dish.

7. Put in the oven preheated to 360 F (180 C) for about 25 minutes.
8. If the top starts browning, gently cover the peppers with aluminum foil.
9. Once ready, set aside for 5 minutes and then serve with the garlic sauce. Enjoy!

- **Dinner**: Let's have delicious almond turkey!

Serves: 2-3
Ingredients:

- 0.9 lbs. (400g) turkey breast, cut against the grain into inch slices
- 1 egg
- 3.5 oz. (100 g) almond flakes
- a tiny pinch cayenne pepper
- salt, pepper
- olive oil

Directions:
1. Pound the meat and cut into smaller pieces.

2. Season with salt, black pepper and cayenne pepper, roll in beaten egg and almond flakes.

3. Preheat the oil in the skillet. You can add a little bit of natural grass-fed butter to taste. Add turkey and fry the meat on both sides.

4. Serve with lettuce and cherry tomato halves (season with salt, drizzle with olive oil and lemon juice).

Conclusion

I want to thank you for buying this book and the time that you have invested in reading it. I hope that I was able to help provide you with all the essential information that you need to keep yourself healthy and fit.

Anti-inflammatory diets are easy to get right once you are well versed in the basics. Through my eBook, the impetus has been on providing you with a reliable data resource that can answer all the doubts and questions you ever had about anti-inflammatory diets. I hope you found all the answers you were seeking.

Finally, if you enjoyed this book, I would really appreciate your review on Amazon!

Thank you again and I wish you great health!

Recommended Reading For You:
You may also want to check my other books:

<u>Gluten-Free Vegan Cookbook: 90+ Healthy, Easy and Delicious Recipes for Vegan Breakfasts, Salads, Soups, Lunches, Dinners and Desserts</u>

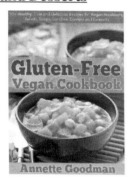

90+ Healthy, Easy and Delicious Recipes for Vegan Breakfasts, Salads, Soups, Lunches, Dinners and Desserts for Your Well-Being + Shopping List to Save Your Precious Time

Gluten-Free Vegan diet doesn't have to be bland and boring at all! These recipes are original, easy to make and just delightfully appetizing. They will enrich your culinary experience and let you enjoy your breakfasts, lunches, dinners and desserts with your friends and family.

In this book you will find:

-23 Scrumptious and Easy Breakfasts

-27 Delicious and Savoury Lunches and Dinners

-22 Aromatic And Nutritious Soups

-21 Enticing And Rich Desserts

-Extra Shopping List to Save Your Precious Time

= 93 Fantastic Gluten-Free Healthy Vegan Recipes!

The Gluten-Free diet will help you detoxify, improve your immune system and make you feel younger - both mentally and physically! The Change is just in front of you!

-> Direct Buy Link:
http://www.amazon.com/dp/B00LU915YA/

-> Paperback Version:
https://www.createspace.com/4907669

Fast Freezer Meals: 46 Delicious and Quick Gluten-Free Slow Cooker Recipes for Make-Ahead Meals That Will Save Your Time and Improve Your Health

Discover Delicious and Quick Gluten-Free Slow Cooker Recipes for Make-Ahead Meals That Will Save Your Time and Improve Your Health!

As a busy businesswoman, wife and mom I know exactly how hard it is to

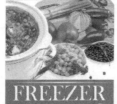
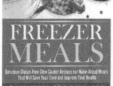

prepare healthy and tasty meals for me and my family every day, especially when they have to be gluten-free! See yourself that gluten-diet doesn't have to be bland, and home cooking doesn't have to be time-consuming!

Most of these recipes can be prepared in no more than 30 minutes and then just effortlessly cooked in your crockpot when you're at work or doing your business!

-I included a shopping list inside to save your precious time.

-No matter if you are gluten intolerant or not – these meals are delicious, healthy and suitable for everyone!

-In this book you will also find freezing and thawing safety guide. These recipes will enrich your culinary experience and let you save massive time!

-> **Direct Buy Link:** http://www.amazon.com/dp/B00M783PS2/

-> **Paperback Version:** https://www.createspace.com/4944068

Paleo Smoothie Recipes: 67 Delicious Paleo Smoothies for Weight Loss and a Healthy Lifestyle

67 Easy and Fast Delicious Smoothie Recipes for Effective Weight Loss and Sexy Body!

Kill the food cravings and get in shape with these delicious and healthy Paleo Smoothies!

In This Book I'll Show You:

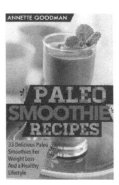

-Why Paleo Smoothies are great for Weight Loss (and Weight Maintenance!)

-67 Tasty Paleo Recipes great for Weight Loss, Detox, and keeping your body Healthy every day! -How to make the Paleo approach easier!

-Important facts about some of the ingredients you'd like to know.

-Planning and Directions – how to get started fast!
-How to maintain your motivation, finally lose the extra pounds and be happy with a Sexy Body!

->**Direct Buy Link:** http://www.amazon.com/dp/B00J8ZHMIQ/

->**Paperback Version:** https://www.createspace.com/4803901

Gluten Free Crock Pot Recipes: 59 Healthy, Easy and Delicious Slow Cooker Paleo Recipes for Breakfast, Lunch and Dinner

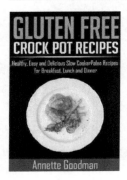

Discover Healthy, Easy and Delicious Slow Cooker Paleo Recipes for Breakfast, Lunch and Dinner for You and Your Family!

Save your time and start healthy living with these delectable slow cooker gluten free recipes tailor-made for busy people!

I've been on the Gluten Free diet for more than ten years now! Although the main reason for my radical diet change was my diagnosis (Coeliac disease), I would never-ever (even if given a magical chance) take the lane of eating gluten again!

-> **Direct Buy Link:** http://www.amazon.com/dp/B00K5UVYUA/

-> **Paperback Version:** https://www.createspace.com/4823966

Low Carb Slow Cooker: 50 Delicious, Fast and Easy Crock Pot Recipes for Rapid Weight Loss

Start Losing Weight Effectively and For Good!

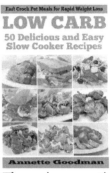

The recipes mentioned in this book are not only simple but they require every day ingredients from your kitchen.

Food tastes best when you cook it with some love. Nothing can beat the mouth-watering dishes that can be cooked in a slow cooker.

If you often find yourself confused about how to whip up a yummy dish for a low-carb diet, this book is just the perfect thing you need right now.

In This Book You Will Read About:

-What is Low Carb Diet?

-Who Should Use it And Who Should Not?

-Pros and Properties of Low Carb Diet

-Some Common Low Carb Myths

-Best and Worst Food Choices You Can Make

-Foods You Need to Avoid

-Important Tips and Advice

-10 Low-Carb Slow-Cooker Aromatic Soups Recipes

-11 Low-Carb Crockpot Delicious Chicken recipes

-10 Low-carb Slow-cooker Amazingly Good Sea-food

-10 Low-carb slow-cooker Yummy Pork Recipes

-9 Low-carb Slow-cooker Scrumptious Lamb Recipes

-> Direct Buy Link: http://www.amazon.com/dp/B00O2AACR0/

-> Paperback Version: https://www.createspace.com/5042178

You may also want to download my friend's books.

Help your mind today with these:

- Buddhism: Beginner's Guide:

  http://www.amazon.com/dp/B00MHSR5YM/

- Meditation: Beginner's Guide:

  http://www.amazon.com/ dp/B00KQRU9BC/

- Zen: Beginner's Guide:

  http://www.amazon.com/dp/B00PWUBSEK/

My Mailing list: If you would like to **receive new Kindle reads** on **weight loss, wellness, diets, recipes and healthy living** for **FREE** I invite you to my Mailing List. Whenever my new book is out, I set the free period for two days. You will get an e-mail notification and will **be the first to get the book for $0** during its limited promotion.

Why would I do this when it took me countless hours to write these e-books?

First of all, that's my way of saying **"thank you"** to my new readers. Second of all – **I want to spread the word about my new books and ideas.** Mind you that **I hate spam and e-mails that come too frequently** - no worries about that.

If you think that's a good idea and are in, just follow this link:

http://eepurl.com/6elQD

You can also follow us on Facebook:

www.facebook.com/HolisticWellnessBooks

We have created this page with a few fellow authors of mine. We hope you find it inspiring and helpful.

Thank You for your time and interest in our work!

Annette Goodman & Holistic Wellness eBooks

About The Author

Hello! My name is Annette Goodman.

I'm glad we met. Who am I?

A homegrown cook, successful wellness aficionado and a writer. I live in Portland, Oregon with my husband, son and our dear golden retriever, Fluffy. I work as a retail manager in of the European companies.

My entire childhood I suffered from obesity, hypertension and complexion problems. During my college years I decided to turn my life around and started my weight-loss and wellness pursue. After more than a decade I can say that I definitely succeeded and now I'd like to give you a hand.

I love creating new healthy recipes, cooking and writing books about healthy lifestyle for you to enjoy and profit from.

I hope we'll meet again!

My Amazon author page:

http://www.amazon.com/Annette-Goodman/e/B00LLPE1QM/

19770947R00044

Made in the USA
San Bernardino, CA
11 March 2015